NOURISH AND FLOURISH

Kid-Tested and Approved Tips and Recipes to Prevent Diabetes

Nancy L. Heinrich, M.P.H.

DEDICATION

To my son, Edward Eddowes*.

Your profound love of music inspires me every day.

*Member, Vero Beach High School Jazz Band, Vero Beach, FL 2009-2012

Member, Vero Beach High School Marching Band, Vero Beach, FL 2008-2012

Member, Vero Beach High School Symphonic Band, Vero Beach, FL 2009-2012

Member, Vero Beach High School Symphonic Band I at Carnegie Hall, New York, NY, 2010

"A jazz musician can improvise based on his knowledge of music. He understands how things go together. For a chef, once you have that basis, that's when cuisine is truly exciting."

~Charlie Trotter

CONTENTS

Acknowledgments 6

1 Your Children's Health 8

2 Breakfast 14

3 Lunch and Snacks 20

4 Dinner Ideas 30

5 Recipe Shopping Lists 50

6 Super Foods 58

7 Family Shopping Lists 60

8 About Growing Healthy Kids 64

9 About the Author 65

ACKNOWLEDGMENTS

I am forever grateful to those individuals who support our work to educate parents about protecting their children from obesity-related diseases such as diabetes. To Ella Chabot-Policare for seeing the vision of the Growing Healthy Kids movement from the very beginning, for her creativity, for listening to me, and for her friendship. To Barbara Petrillo for collaborating to raise awareness about our work and our mission. To Ginny Rhodes at Youth Guidance Mentoring & Activities Program for coordinating each of the amazing educational events we have conducted for kids in need of mentors. To Janie Hoover-Graves for responding to my request for book title suggestions with her three words: "Nourish and Flourish". To the thousands of children who have asked for seconds and thirds at our Growing Healthy Kids in the Kitchen programs and Giant Salad Parties for their energy and their eagerness to learn about eating real whole foods. To the parents who have said to me, "I've never seen my son (or daughter) eat vegetables like this before your class," for teaching me that we must actively educate you if we are going to reverse the childhood obesity epidemic in America. To the parents in America who want to know what to do if your child is at an unhealthy weight for making the decision to stop being embarrassed and do something about it. To my mother, Anna Wilson, for always being there for me and for believing in me. To my brothers, William and Robert, for your unwavering support.

This book is inspired by the children who have been part of the "Growing Healthy Kids in the Kitchen and the Garden" educational programs at Vero Beach Elementary School, Hibiscus Children's Center, Dasie Hope Center, The Willow School, Youth Guidance Mentoring & Activities Program, and Boys & Girls Clubs of Indian River County. With your energy, your enthusiasm, and your willingness to taste new flavors and foods, I am confident that we can reverse, halt, and prevent childhood obesity in this country. Now, let's teach your parents!

With love,
Nancy L. Heinrich, M.P.H.
Founder, Growing Healthy Kids, Inc.

CHAPTER 1

YOUR CHILDREN'S HEALTH

What's so bad about sugar and corn syrup? A lot, if you eat too much. Excess sugar consumption is linked not only to obesity, but also to kidney stones, osteoporosis, heart disease, and dental cavities. Sugar and corn syrup are also addictive – the more you eat, the more you want. Plus, the more sugar and other empty calories you eat, the more other calories you have to eat just to get your minimum daily requirement of vitamins and other nutritional factors.

~ John Robbins

Nourish. Flourish. These two words describe the **Growing Healthy Kids** movement to prevent obesity-related diseases like diabetes and heart disease in children. "Nourish" means to provide someone or something with food and other things that are needed to live and be healthy. "Flourish" means to grow well, to be healthy. Kids need real foods to be healthy and live well. Think of this book as your parent manual.

As an epidemiologist and diabetes educator, I have heard hundreds of adults say to me, "I wish I would have known what you are teaching me when I saw a kid. Then I wouldn't have diabetes now." We know that obesity is the primary risk factor for developing type 2 diabetes. Give the dramatic increase in obesity in the U.S. in the past 20 years and the fact that **one in three children in American is overweight or obese**, I started the Growing Healthy Kids organization to teach kids and parents about simple ways to get to – and stay at – healthier weights and prevent obesity-related diseases including diabetes.

If children are overweight and obese, then obesity in adulthood is likely to be more severe. Since 1980, obesity prevalence among children and adolescents ages 2-19 has almost tripled. I believe it is important for all adults who can influence the food and physical activity choices made by children to understand the consequences of obesity. According to Centers for Disease Control and Prevention, obese children are more likely to have:

- High blood pressure and high cholesterol which are risk factors for cardiovascular disease

- Increased risk of impaired glucose tolerance, insulin resistance, and type 2 diabetes (often called "adult-onset diabetes")

- Breathing problems such as sleep apnea and asthma

- Joint problems and musculoskeletal discomfort

- Fatty liver disease, gallstones, and gastro-esophageal reflux (i.e., heartburn)

- Greater risk of social and psychosocial problems such as discrimination and poor self-esteem which can continue into adulthood

Sometimes kids attending their first "Growing Healthy Kids in the Kitchen" program say, "I don't think I'm going to like this" when they see a sea of fresh vegetables in front of them. After we've made a recipe together and everyone has had a taste, their words transform into "Wow, this is delicious!" "You've got to try this!" and "I can't wait to make this at home."

Maybe it's because I'm not their mom nagging them to "eat your vegetables." Maybe it's the fact that we have fun learning about new foods, chopping vegetables together, and learning how to prepare foods that taste good AND are good for you. The fact is when you eat whole, real foods, your kids perform better at school, you perform better at work, you and your kids have more energy for sports, and everyone feels better every day and sleeps better every night.

The recipes and tips in NOURISH AND FLOURISH are plant-based. They have been selected from our expanding collection of kid-tested and approved foods. Best of all, they taste great, are easy and inexpensive to make, and are good for you and your kids.

Ask your child's pediatrician what they would like to change about what kids eat. They will tell you it is to help kids avoid foods high in sugar, fat, and calories, stay at healthy weights, and avoid developing obesity-related adult diseases such as diabetes and high blood pressure. Use this book as a guide to keep highly processed, high calorie, high fat and sugar-filled foods out of your family's kitchen.

Here are two rules to get you started:

Growing Healthy Kids Rule #1 is HAVE FUN! Have fun exploring the tips and recipes in this book. Have fun learning about foods that taste great and keep you healthy. Have fun introducing your children to the farmers at your local green market. Have fun adding "super foods" to your grocery lists. Have fun teaching your kids how to cut up an apple. Have fun reading and using this book because NOURISH AND FLOURISH is about great foods for Growing Healthy Kids – in this case, your own children!

Growing Healthy Kids Rule #2 is EAT RAINBOWS! Choose vegetables and fruits that are the colors of rainbows: red, yellow, green, purple, orange, and blue.

The fact is that eating real foods in the right amounts, combined with regular physical activity, is key to getting to and staying at a healthy weight for the rest of your life. Wherever the Growing Healthy Kids' programs go, what follows is that kids begin craving real foods that fuel a lifetime of strong and healthy bodies and minds. Kids need and deserve access to great foods as their foundation to be strong, smart, and healthy for life. Teaching kids -- and the parents, teachers, principals, cafeteria managers, and afterschool program staff who surround them -- how to grow, prepare, and enjoy delicious, healthy meals and snacks and to enjoy physical activity *every day* is what we do. In this book parents will learn this lesson: **when you know what to do, it's easy!**

Here is a story about why our Growing Healthy Kids movement has been become so powerful. Recently I showed up at the local Boys & Girls Club. The kids were so excited about the prospect of what they were going to learn that they literally *stormed the front door* of the club when they saw my car pull into the parking lot. Staff had to quickly redirect them - and their excitement. But you know what? The staff saw how excited the kids were because they also knew the magic of healthy eating was about to begin as I walked through the door with a cooler full of just-picked, fresh vegetables and flavorful herbs. The staff knew they would soon be sampling recipes containing foods like blueberries and walnuts with delicious flavors to help them get to healthier weights and prevent diabetes that some of them were already facing. You know what? The staff at the Boys & Girls Club would have stormed the door, too, *if the kids wouldn't have been watching!*

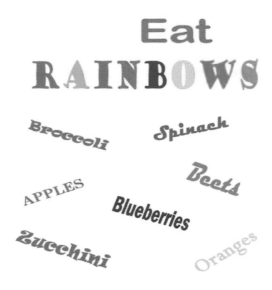

ASSESSMENT QUESTIONS

HOW MANY DAYS A WEEK I EXERCISE AT LEAST 30 MINUTES:

HOW MANY HOURS OF SLEEP I GET MOST NIGHTS:

MY FAVORITE FRUIT:

MY FAVORITE VEGETABLE:

MY FAVORITE GRAIN:

WHAT I DRINK MOST OFTEN:

ONE THING I WOULD LIKE TO EAT LESS OF:

ONE THING I WOULD LIKE TO IMPROVE ABOUT WHAT I EAT IS:

HOW MANY DAYS A WEEK MY CHILD EXERCISES AT LEAST 60 MINUTES:

HOW MANY HOURS OF SLEEP MY CHILD GETS MOST NIGHTS:

MY CHILD'S FAVORITE FRUIT:

MY CHILD'S FAVORITE VEGETABLE:

MY CHILD'S FAVORITE GRAIN:

WHAT MY CHILD DRINKS MOST OFTEN:

ONE THING I WOULD LIKE MY CHILD TO EAT LESS OF IS:

ONE THING I WOULD LIKE TO IMPROVE ABOUT WHAT MY CHILD EATS IS:

CHAPTER 2

BREAKFAST

"When you wake up in the morning, Pooh,' said Piglet at last, 'what's the first thing you say to yourself?' 'What's for breakfast?' said Pooh. 'What do you say, Piglet?' 'I say, I wonder what's going to happen exciting today,' said Piglet. Pooh nodded thoughtfully, 'It's the same thing,' he said."

~A.A. Milne, <u>The House at Pooh Corner</u>

GROWING HEALTHY KIDS: Our Recipe Collection
Fabulous Fruit Shakes

BLEND in a blender:

- 1 cup almond milk* OR fat-free milk
- 1 cup frozen fruit (such as blueberries, bananas, strawberries, mangos)
- 1 teaspoon ground flax seeds
- 1 teaspoon vanilla (optional)
- Dash of ground cinnamon (optional)

*For demonstration purposes, Blue Diamond Almond Milk (1 cup has 60 calories) was used in the preparation of this recipe.

GROWING HEALTHY KIDS TIP #1:

Eat a variety of fruit every day for strong bodies and great health. Blueberries, strawberries, and bananas, three of the world's healthiest fruits, are nutritious, and taste great.

Blueberries are low in calories (40 calories per half cup) and are powerful disease fighters. They contain fiber and vitamin C. These little berries are powerful disease fighters and may prevent memory diseases and some forms of cancer. Fresh or frozen blueberries are both great choices.

Strawberries are the most popular berry in the U.S. They are very low in calories (20 calories per half cup). They are rich in antioxidants plus heart-healthy nutrients and are an excellent source of vitamin C.

Bananas are a great source of potassium which helps keep our blood pressure at healthy levels. Other foods that contain potassium include tomatoes, oranges, and dates.

GROWING HEALTHY KIDS: Our Recipe Collection

Pecan Pancakes with a Burst of Blueberries

BLEND in a blender:

- ½ to 1/3 cup of pecans
- 3-½ cups quick cooking oats
- 4 cups water
- 2 teaspoons vanilla
- 1 teaspoon sea salt
- 2 Tablespoons honey or agave nectar

POUR into large bowl.

ADD 1-½ cups of blueberries.

COOK on nonstick griddle or skillet.

SERVE with nonfat vanilla yogurt, agave nectar and a sprinkle of cinnamon.

GROWING HEALTHY KIDS TIP #2:

Take time to enjoy your meals. When you eat a meal in less than 20 minutes, your stomach does not have enough time to send the following message up to your brain, "We've got enough food for now. Stop sending the 'I'm starving' signals."

Eating too fast and eating too much food can lead to indigestion or an upset stomach.   Just like you plan a grocery list based on your family's menus, plan relaxed family meals several times a week. Plan a leisurely family breakfast at least once a week.

GROWING HEALTHY KIDS: Our Recipe Collection
Super Oats

BRING TO A BOIL:
- 3 cups water

ADD:
- 1 cup steel cut oats
- ¼ teaspoon sea salt

REDUCE heat to a low simmer.

COVER AND COOK for 10 minutes ("al dente") to 20 minutes (creamy).

STIR several times.

REMOVE from heat and let stand for 2 minutes.

MAKES 4 servings.

SERVING SUGGESTIONS:
- Almond milk
- Brown sugar or agave nectar
- Fresh or frozen blueberries
- Craisins or dried cherries
- Chopped walnuts
- Cinnamon
- Ground flax seed

TIP: This recipe refrigerates well for super easy, super healthy, and super inexpensive school and work day breakfasts. One serving of cooked steel cut oats (1/4 cup of dry oats) contains 170 calories, 5 grams of dietary fiber (including 1.6 grams of soluble fiber), and 7 grams of protein and costs 27 cents.

*For demonstration purposes, Bob's Red Mill Steel Cut Oats were used in the preparation of this recipe.

GROWING HEALTHY KIDS TIP #3:

Drink water not soda.

Water is what our bodies need and crave but most people don't drink enough. Flavor water with fresh lime or lemon juice or slices of cucumber or watermelon. Avoid or limit sodas because most sodas contain high fructose corn syrup, a highly processed sugar that contributes to weight gain. Drinking plenty of water helps fill you up and keeps your skin healthy. If you drink an eight ounce glass once an hour during the day you can easily get enough of this precious fluid.

NOTES:

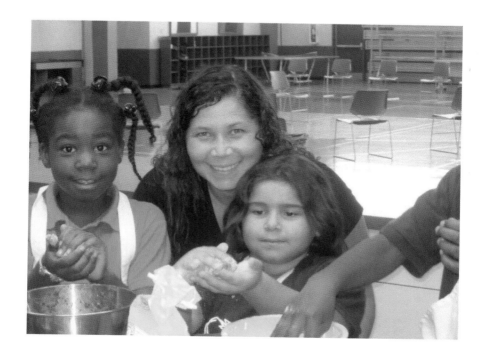

Parents and kids learning together at a "Growing Healthy Kids in the Kitchen" event.

CHAPTER 3

LUNCH AND SNACKS

**In general, mankind, since the improvement in cookery,
eats twice as much as nature requires.**

~Benjamin Franklin

GROWING HEALTHY KIDS: Our Recipe Collection
Garden Pizza

SLICE:

- Baby Bella mushrooms
- Sun-dried tomatoes or Roma tomatoes
- Other veggies such as fresh spinach, red and green peppers, onions, black olives

SAUTE mushrooms in a small pan with:

- extra virgin olive oil
- chopped garlic

SAUTE in a medium saucepan for 5-10 minutes:

- 3 cloves garlic, chopped
- 1 Tablespoon each dried basil and oregano
- 2 Tablespoons extra virgin olive oil
- 1 can no-salt added tomato paste
- ¾ to 1 cup water (enough for "pizza sauce" consistency)

SPREAD pizza sauce on a flat bread*:

SPRINKLE vegetables on flatbread.

TOP with:

- ½ cup mozzarella cheese

BAKE at 375 degrees for about 10 minutes.

*For demonstration purposes, **Tandoori Whole-Grain Naan** flatbreads (170 calories and 4 grams of dietary fiber per ½ Naan) were used in the preparation of this recipe.

Let kids build their own pizzas with their choice of toppings. Have a "Build Your Own Pizza Night" once a week. Create personalized invitations and ask your kids to invite a friend over for extra fun!

More pizza topping ideas:

- Pineapple, eggplant, broccoli
- Morningstar Farms sausage or bacon strips
- Feta cheese, caramelized onions

GROWING HEALTHY KIDS TIP #4:

Use herbs to season foods. Herbs such as basil, oregano, parsley, cilantro, and thyme are easy to grow and add flavor, color, and variety.

Start your own "kitchen garden" and keep a pot of your favorite herbs using recycled containers with a couple of holes cut, punched, or drilled in the bottom.

NOTE FROM NANCY: Adult supervision may be needed with this activity.

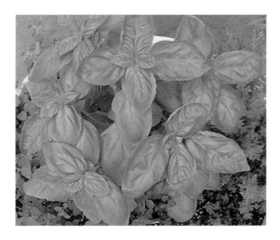

GROWING HEALTHY KIDS: Our Recipe Collection
PB&Bs*

LAY ON PLATE:

- 1 slice whole grain bread**

TOP WITH:

- 1-2 Tablespoons natural peanut butter* or almond butter
- ½ banana, sliced
- 5-6 raisins (optional)

*Peanut Butter and Banana

For demonstration purposes, Arnold's Flax & Fiber bread (because it meets "The Nancy Rule" – see Tip 9 on page 32) and Smucker's Creamy Natural Peanut Butter (because it contains no added sugar or fats**) were used in the preparation of this recipe.

GROWING HEALTHY KIDS TIP #5:

Become a sugar detective.   Choose foods and drinks without added sugars. Why? Sugar has many names and it is hidden in common foods that we eat every day.

Here are some of the names for sugar in packaged and processed foods:

1. Agave nectar

2. Barbados sugar

3. Barley malt

4. Beet sugar

5. Blackstrap molasses

6. Brown sugar

7. Buttered sugar

8. Cane crystals

9. Cane juice crystals

10. Cane sugar

11. Caramel

12. Carob syrup

13. Castor sugar

14. Confectioner's sugar

15. Corn syrup

16. Corn sweetener

17. Corn syrup solids

18. Crystalline fructose

19. Date sugar

20. Dextrin

21. Dextrose

22. Diastatic malt

23. Diastase

24. D-mannose

25. Florida crystals

26. Fructose

27. Fruit juice

28. Fruit juice concentrates

NOTES:

29. Galactose

30. Glucose

31. Glucose solids

32. Golden sugar

33. Golden syrup

34. Granulated sugar

35. Grape sugar

36. Grape juice concentrate

37. HFCS

38. HMCS

39. High fructose corn syrup

40. High maltose corn syrup

41. Honey

42. Invert sugar

43. Lactose

44. Malt syrup

45. Maltodextrin

46. Maltose

47. Mannitol

48. Maple syrup

49. Molasses

50. Organic raw sugar

51. Powdered sugar

TIP FOR READING FOOD LABELS:

If a breakfast cereal or granola bar has more than 8 grams of sugar per serving (which is 2 teaspoons of sugar), then don't buy it. Choose one with less sugar, not more.

52. Raw sugar

53. Rice syrup

54. Sorbitol

55. Sorghum syrup

56. Sucrose

57. Sugar

58. Table sugar

59. Turbinado sugar

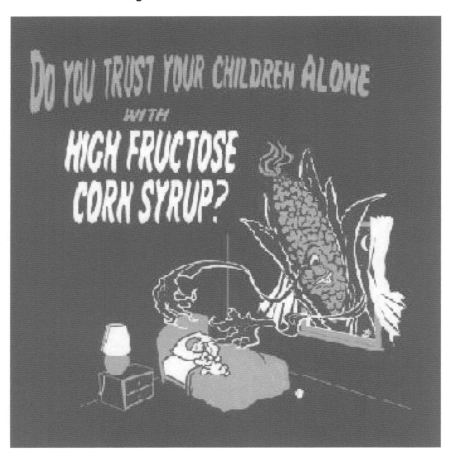

GROWING HEALTHY KIDS: Our Recipe Collection
Wrap It!

WHISK in a large bowl:
- 3 Tablespoons extra virgin olive oil
- 1 Tablespoon red wine vinegar

SEASON with:
- Sea salt
- Fresh ground black pepper

MIX into the dressing:
- 1-1/4 cups chopped plum or cherry or grape tomatoes
- 1 cup diced and peeled cucumbers
- 1 cup chopped green bell peppers
- ½ cup chopped radishes
- 2/3 cup chopped red onion
- ½ cup chopped fresh flat leaf parsley

STIR in:
- 1 cup crumbled feta cheese
  (about 4-1/2 ounces)

USE a slotted spoon to transfer salad into:
- Four 8-inch-diameter whole wheat pita breads, cut in half

SERVE immediately.

GROWING HEALTHY KIDS TIP #6:

Kids AND adults need vegetables every day. Vegetables contain dietary fiber (which is only found in plant foods that grow from the Earth) which helps fill us up so we don't eat too much. Make it your goal to eat more vegetables than fruit every day.

GROWING HEALTHY KIDS: Our Recipe Collection
Hummus

PLACE in food processor or blender and mix together:
- One 16-ounce can garbanzo beans, drained and rinsed
- 2 Tablespoons tahini (sesame seed butter)
- 3-5 Tablespoons lemon juice
- 3 garlic cloves, crushed
- 1 Tablespoon extra virgin olive oil (or 5-6 black olives)
- 1/4 teaspoon sea salt

STORAGE: 3 days in the fridge or 1 month in the freezer.

OTHER FLAVORS to make:
- Artichoke-lemon hummus: Add 1 cup marinated artichoke hearts and an extra ¼ cup lemon juice.
- Sun-dried tomato hummus: Add ½ cup sun-dried tomatoes.

CHOP 2 or 3 of your favorite vegetables, such as tomatoes, peppers, and cucumbers.

SERVE hummus for lunch in a whole grain pita or wrap or as a snack with the veggies:
- Use whole grain pitas or wraps with 4 or more grams of dietary fiber per serving.
- Use whole grain crackers with 4 or more grams of dietary fiber per serving.

GROWING HEALTHY KIDS TIP #7: **Garbanzos and other beans are a great source of dietary fiber, with about 5-6 grams per ½ cup.** Eating high fiber and whole grain foods for snacks and meals fills you up and prevents you from overeating. If you have diabetes or prediabetes, eating high fiber foods like garbanzo, black, or pinto beans and whole grains like brown rice helps control your blood sugar.

GROWING HEALTHY KIDS: Our Recipe Collection
Success Snacks

COMBINE in a bowl:

- ½ cup dried cherries or cranberries
- ½ cup pistachios, shelled
- ½ cup walnuts
- 2 cups Kashi Heart to Heart cereal with oat flakes and blueberry clusters or Cheerios
- dark chocolate, broken into small pieces (optional)

PUT ½ cup of success snack mix into a snack size zip-lock bag. Makes 8 snack bags.

CREATE your own favorite success snacks with other dried fruits and nuts such as dried apricots, raisins, almonds, and cashews.

GROWING HEALTHY KIDS TIP #8:

Healthy snacks should include a little fruit and/or vegetables plus something with a little protein and fat. Add a reduced-fat string cheese or a fat-free Greek yogurt with your Success Snack to make this a great after-school snack.

MORE HEALTHY SNACK IDEAS FOR KIDS OF ALL AGES:

- 3-4 walnut halves and half a banana or peach
- half a pear or apple and a couple of slices of your favorite cheddar cheese
- sliced cucumbers and ¼ cup hummus
- fat-free yogurt sprinkled with ground flax seed

CHAPTER 4

DINNER IDEAS

It's difficult to think anything but pleasant thoughts while eating a homegrown tomato.

~Lewis Grizzard

GROWING HEALTHY KIDS: Our Recipe Collection
Favorite Tomato Sauce

BLANCH:

- 3 pounds ripe tomatoes (or use 2 28-oz cans of whole, plum tomatoes, save the juice for use if the sauce needs thinning). Cut an "X" on the bottom of the tomato, then drop in boiling water for 30 seconds. Holding tomatoes over a bowl, peel, and core them.

CHOP tomatoes roughly and set aside. Strain juices from bowl; add half of the juices to the chopped tomatoes. Save or freeze the other half for recipes that call for tomato juice.

HEAT in a fry pan or pot for 30 seconds:

- 1/4 cup extra virgin olive oil

ADD and stir for 30 seconds after adding each ingredient:

- Pinch of sea salt
- 8 cloves garlic, chopped
- ½ teaspoon hot pepper flakes

ADD and cook while stirring until boiling:

- Chopped tomatoes and juices

ADD:

- 1-1/2 Tablespoons dried basil (if using dried basil)
- 1 Tablespoon balsamic vinegar
- 6 sun-dried tomatoes, chopped finely

MIX WELL and reduce heat to medium-low.

COOK for 20-25 minutes, stirring occasionally.

ADD and continue cooking for 5 minutes:

- ¼-1/2 cup fresh basil, packed down (if using fresh basil)

REMOVE from heat, cover, and let "rest" for 5-10 minutes to develop flavor.

STIR and serve over pasta*.

*For demonstration purposes, Barilla Whole Grain Spaghetti with 6 grams of dietary fiber per serving was used in the preparation of this recipe.

This recipe makes 4 cups of sauce, enough for pasta to serve 8. Use this for any recipe calling for tomato sauce, such as lasagna, baked ziti, and spaghetti. It freezes well and is easy to make in large batches.

GROWING HEALTHY KIDS TIP #9:

CHOOSE whole grain spaghetti that meets "The Nancy Rule":   4 or more grams of dietary fiber per serving AND the first ingredient includes the word "whole" as in "whole grain".

USE "The Nancy Rule" to get enough dietary fiber (key to preventing and controlling diabetes because fiber is the "good" carbohydrate). In addition to spaghetti and other types of pasta, use "The Nancy Rule" as a guideline for choosing breads, flatbreads, tortillas, and crackers.

TIP: Teach this rule to your kids and give them the job of using it when they go food shopping with you. Show them where to find "fiber" under "total carbohydrates" on food labels. Remember, fiber is the good kind of carbohydrate, sugar is the bad kind.

GROWING HEALTHY KIDS: Our Recipe Collection

Pesto

BLEND in a blender:

- 3-4 garlic cloves
- ¼ cup walnuts (about 7 or 8 walnut halves)
- ¾ cup grated parmesan cheese
- 2 cups fresh basil leaves, loosely packed
- ¾ cup extra virgin olive oil

SERVE on whole grain pasta and your favorite grilled or sautéed vegetables.

A DELICIOUS PESTO IDEA: Make a Mediterranean pizza. Use pesto as the sauce on whole grain Naan flatbread or a whole grain muffin. Add feta cheese, sliced olives, and sundried tomatoes. Top with mozzarella cheese and bake at 350 degrees for about 10 minutes. Serve with fresh grated parmesan cheese.

GROWING HEALTHY KIDS TIP #10:

Most of the fat we eat should be the "good" fats, called unsaturated fats: fish, nuts (like walnuts and almonds), olives, avocados, flax seeds, and liquid vegetable oils like extra virgin olive oil.

Limit the "bad" fats you eat. These are called **saturated fats** (found in meat, cheese, butter and other foods from animals) and **trans fats** (see *Growing Healthy Kids Tip #13*).

GROWING HEALTHY KIDS: Our Recipe Collection
Pico De Gallo
(pronounced "pee-co day guy-yo")

COMBINE in a bowl:

- 2 medium tomatoes, cut into ¼-inch cubes
- ¼ cup finely diced red onion
- 1 jalapeño pepper, finely diced (with or without seeds, depending on desired hotness) (ADULTS) OR
- ½ green pepper, finely diced (KIDS)
- ½ teaspoon sea salt
- fresh lime juice from 2 limes

ADD:

- 1 Tablespoon extra virgin olive oil (optional)
- 2 Tablespoons fresh cilantro, finely chopped

TRANSFER to a serving bowl. Let rest for about 1 hour, covered and unrefrigerated, for best flavor. This is great served with whole grain chips or on enchiladas and quesadillas.

NOTE: Use gloves if working with jalapeño peppers. DO NOT rub your eyes.

GROWING HEALTHY KIDS TIP #11: **Eat dinner together.**
A new national study led by epidemiologist Sarah Anderson at Ohio State University analyzed data on 8,550 4-year olds and found that children who practiced 2 healthy lifestyle behaviors were slimmer than those who adopted only one behavior, while youngsters who implemented three beneficial habits were the least likely to be overweight. According to Sarah, "If children had all 3 routines, their risk of obesity was 40% lower than children who had none of the routines." Know what the 3 habits were? Eating dinner regularly with family, limiting the time spent in front of the TV, and getting enough sleep.

GROWING HEALTHY KIDS: Our Recipe Collection

Garden Quinoa

(Pronunciation guide: Gar-den Keen-Wha)

What is Quinoa? Quinoa is a grain. It is the only grain that is a complete protein. You have to rinse it before you cook it to remove the bitter coating that protects the grain so birds don't eat it. Put quinoa in a sieve and shake it under running water for 1-2 minutes.*

Ingredients:

- 1½ cups low-sodium chicken stock, vegetable broth, or water
- 1 cup quinoa, thoroughly rinsed and drained*
- ½ teaspoon salt
- ½ teaspoon black pepper
- 1 cup frozen chopped, mixed vegetables such as peas, carrots, green beans, corn

Directions:

ADD: chicken stock or water to medium saucepan. With an adult's help, bring chicken stock or water to a boil over medium-high heat.

STIR in quinoa, salt, and pepper.

TURN heat down to low and cover pot with lid.

COOK till water is evaporated and quinoa is tender, about 15 minutes.

REMOVE lid and stir in veggies with a fork.

PLACE lid back on quinoa so that the heat from the quinoa cooks the vegetables.

SERVE immediately or place into an airtight container and refrigerate for up to 5 days.

NOTE FROM NANCY: This recipe is great served cold for school lunch boxes and work lunches.

GROWING HEALTHY KIDS TIP #12:

Eat fruit. Limit or avoid fruit juice.

Why? Whole fruit contains fiber but juice doesn't. Juice is all sugar and even though it is "fruit sugar" (called fructose), it is still sugar. The fact is that eating too much sugar can make us gain unwanted weight.

Remember that "fresh" and "frozen" fruit are better choices than canned fruit or fruit juices.

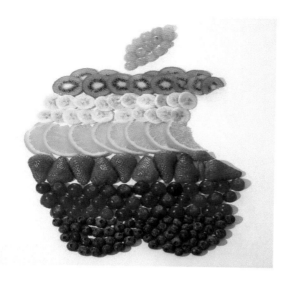

Fill in the blank: "An apple a day_____ _____."

GROWING HEALTHY KIDS: Our Recipe Collection
Guacamole

MASH in a medium bowl with a fork:

- 1 Haas avocado
- Juice of ½ lime or lemon
- 2-3 cloves garlic
- Hot sauce to taste (we like Crystal Hot Sauce)
- ¼ cup chopped cilantro
- Sea salt to taste

SERVE with Pico de Gallo and whole grain chips such as Sun Chips or your favorite corn chips.

GROWING HEALTHY KIDS TIP #13:

Avoid trans fats ("partially hydrogenated" oils).

Why? **The Institute of Medicine has concluded there is NO SAFE LEVEL OF TRANS FATS.** Trans fats raise your bad cholesterol levels.

Beware of hidden trans fats in processed foods. If a food label says "0 trans fat", then look for these 2 words, "partially hydrogenated," on the ingredient list. If you see "partially hydrogenated", then there are small amounts of trans fats in the food.

What food manufacturers don't want you to know is that they are legally allowed by the FDA to add up to ½ gram of trans fat per serving yet claim that it contains none.

GROWING HEALTHY KIDS: Our Recipe Collection

Mashed Cotatoes

Who doesn't like mashed potatoes? This recipe uses cauliflower and it looks and tastes just like mashed potatoes!

CUT UP one head of cauliflower into 2 inch pieces.

STEAM cauliflower in 1 cup of water in a pan, covered with a lid, on medium heat for about 12-15 minutes or until cauliflower is tender with the "fork test".

PUT IN food processor or blender:

- Cauliflower*
- 3 Tablespoons Fleishmann's Olive Oil spread
- 3-4 Tablespoons skim milk
- 1/2 teaspoon sea salt
- Fresh ground pepper

BLEND until cauliflower is the texture of mashed potatoes. Add more milk if necessary.

GROWING HEALTHY KIDS TIP #14:

Did you know......cauliflower is related to cabbage, brussel sprouts, kale, broccoli and collard greens? One cup of raw cauliflower contains about 25 calories, 5 grams of carbohydrates, and 2 grams of dietary fiber.

FACT: Cauliflower contains several phytochemicals which are beneficial to our health, including **sulforaphane**, an anti-cancer compound released when cauliflower is chopped or chewed. In addition, the compound **indole-3-carbinol** appears to slow or prevent the growth of tumors of the breast and prostate.

Eating fresh or frozen vegetables every day is key to great health – yours and your kids.

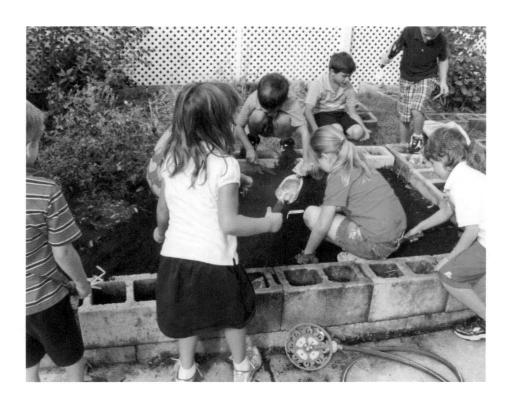

GROWING HEALTHY KIDS: Our Recipe Collection
Frittata with Spinach and Cheese

HEAT in a 9-inch nonstick skillet until hot:
- 2 Tablespoons extra virgin olive oil

ADD in this ingredient and stir until onion is soft, about 5 minutes:
- 1 onion, finely chopped

ADD in these 2 ingredients and cook for about 2 minutes:
- 1 cup spinach, finely chopped
- ¼ cup sun-dried tomatoes, finely chopped OR ½ cup grape tomatoes

MIX these 5 ingredients in a large bowl:
- 8 large eggs
- ¼ cup extra sharp cheese, grated or thinly sliced
- ¼ cup freshly grated parmigiano-reggiano cheese
- Sea salt
- Freshly ground black pepper

POUR egg mixture into the skillet and cook until bottom has set, about 5 minutes.

HOLD a flat plate over the pan and invert frittata onto the plate, then slide it back into the pan. (Note: If you use an oven-proof pan, you can place frittata into oven at 350 degrees for 5 minutes after the bottom has cooked instead of flipping it.)

COOK until just set, about 5 minutes more, and serve hot.

Adapted from a recipe by Mario Batali.

For demonstration purposes, the spinach, tomatoes, and onions used in the preparation of this recipe – and many of the recipes in **Nourish and Flourish** - were purchased on field trips to local farms such as Osceola Organics in Vero Beach, Florida. Whenever possible, use locally grown vegetables from farmers near you.

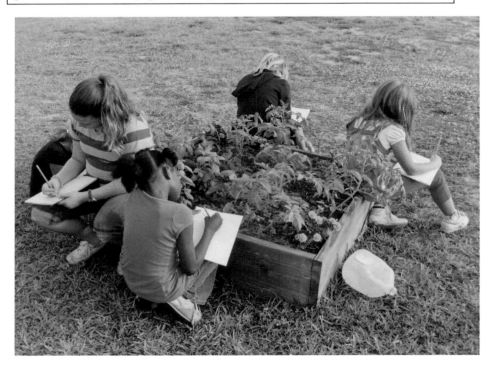

GROWING HEALTHY KIDS TIP #15: **Get to know your local farmers.** Buy "free-range" eggs from local farmers like Linda Hart of Crazy Hart Ranch. Look for Linda selling her free-range eggs year-round at the Saturday morning Green Markets in Vero Beach and Fort Pierce, Florida. Free-range eggs are better than store-bought eggs because they are higher in omega-3 fatty acids and folic acid which are good for brain health and heart health. Eggs are a great, inexpensive source of protein. To locate a farmers market near you, check out www.localharvest.org and www.farmersmarketonline.com.

GROWING HEALTHY KIDS: Our Recipe Collection

Veggie Sloppy Joes

Ingredients:

- ½ cup onions, chopped
- 1 clove garlic, minced
- ½ cup chopped green pepper
- 1 teaspoon extra virgin olive oil
- 1 package Morningstar Farms Grillers Recipe Crumbles
- ½ teaspoon black pepper
- 1 can (8 oz) no-salt added tomato sauce
- 1 cup ketchup (without high fructose corn syrup)
- 1 teaspoon Worcestershire sauce
- 8 whole grain hamburger buns

Directions:

SAUTE onions, garlic, and green pepper in oil in a 2 quart saucepan.

STIR in remaining ingredients (except the buns).

COOK over medium heat, until mixture starts to simmer, stirring occasionally.

REDUCE heat, cover, and simmer 10 minutes.

SERVE hot on hamburger buns. Serves 8.

GROWING HEALTHY KIDS TIP #16:

Fiber is the "good" carbohydrate. This meatless version of the popular Sloppy Joes contains no dietary cholesterol and only 1/2 gram of saturated fat per serving. When you serve these on whole grain buns, you are getting an extra dose of much-needed dietary fiber. The daily goal for fiber is 14 grams of dietary fiber per 1,000 calories. Aim for at least 28 grams of fiber a day.

Most Americans get far less than half the fiber they need. To learn more, check out Dietary Guidelines for Americans 2010 at www.usda.gov. These guidelines are updated once every five years.

GROWING HEALTHY KIDS: Our Recipe Collection

Brain Power Burgers

Ingredients:

- 1 (14.75 ounce) can wild pink salmon, drained
- 1 small can solid albacore tuna packed in water, drained
- 2 teaspoons Dijon mustard
- 1 cup flat-leaf (Italian) parsley, finely chopped
- 1 small yellow onion, finely chopped
- 1 egg
- sea salt and pepper
- 1/2 cup bread crumbs (plus another ½ cup for bowl)

PREHEAT a large pan; spray with nonstick cooking spray.

PLACE salmon, tuna, and Dijon mustard in food processor and pulse briefly until well mixed.

TRANSFER to a large mixing bowl.

ADD remaining ingredients; use a fork to thoroughly combine.

DIVIDE mixture into 6 equal pieces.

FORM burgers into patties. Place about an additional ½ cup bread crumbs in a small bowl. Place formed burgers into bread crumbs and gently pat on both sides.

COOK for about 6-7 minutes, flipping several times, until nicely browned on both sides. Don't overcook! Use cooking spray as needed.

SERVE burgers on whole grain buns. Add a slice of cheese, tomato, and some fresh lettuce or spinach. Top with your favorite condiments such as mustard and chipotle mayo.

GROWING HEALTHY KIDS TIP #17: Wild salmon is considered a "super food" because it is a great source of omega-3 fatty acids and is a source of the "good" fats (unsaturated). Aim for 2 or more servings of fish a week.

GROWING HEALTHY KIDS: Our Recipe Collection

Black Bean Quesadillas

Blend together in blender or food processor (or mash in a large bowl with a fork):

- 1 can cooked black beans, drained and rinsed
- ¼ cup mild salsa

Spread on 4 (of 8) whole wheat tortillas* (can also use corn tortillas):

- 2 Tablespoons shredded cheddar cheese
- black bean mixture

Cover the 4 tortillas with another tortilla.

Grill tortillas in a medium hot nonstick skillet on both sides. Cut each quesadilla into 4 pieces and place on a large platter. Place a small bowl of the salsa in the middle and garnish with fresh sour cream, guacamole, and cilantro.

*For demonstration purposes, **La Tortilla Factory's Smart and Delicious tortillas** were used in the preparation of this recipe. One original size tortilla has 50 calories, 10 total grams of carbohydrates and 7 grams of dietary fiber.

GROWING HEALTHY KIDS TIP #18:

Black beans are an excellent source of dietary fiber. One-half cup of beans provides 7 grams of fiber, 110 calories, and 340 grams of potassium (good for your blood pressure). To get to – and stay at – a healthier weight, choose more foods with dietary fiber to fill you up.

GROWING HEALTHY KIDS: Our Recipe Collection
Pasta with Walnuts

SAUTE in a medium sauté pan for 4-5 minutes:

- 4 cloves garlic, crushed
- 1/3 cup extra virgin olive oil
- ½ cup thinly sliced yellow onions
- 1 cup thinly sliced sweet red pepper

ADD the next ingredients and sauté for another minute:

- 1/8 teaspoon dried red pepper flakes
- ¾ cup finely chopped walnuts
- 2 Tablespoons chopped fresh flat (Italian) parsley
- sea salt and fresh ground pepper to taste

BOIL until al dente in lightly salted water:

- ¾ pound whole grain penne pasta

DRAIN the pasta and return it to the pot. Add the walnut mixture and toss together.

SERVE with freshly grated Parmesan cheese.

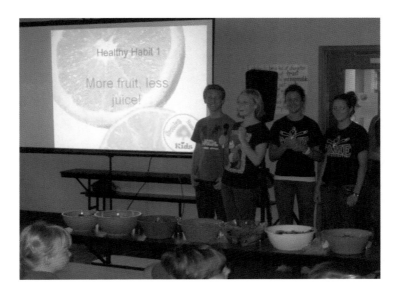

GROWING HEALTHY KIDS TIP #19: Kids (and parents) need vegetables every day. Why? Foods like vegetables and whole grains like brown rice and quinoa contain dietary fiber (only found in plant foods that grow from the Earth) which helps fill us up so we don't eat too much. Make it your goal to eat more vegetables than fruit every day. Have colors at every meal. EAT YOUR RAINBOWS.

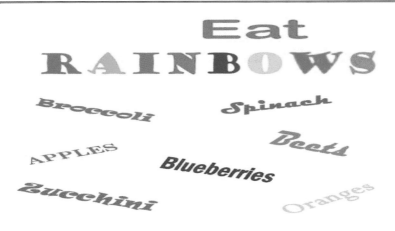

GROWING HEALTHY KIDS: Our Recipe Collection

Veggie Shepherd's Pie

PIE:

SAUTÈ in a medium sauce pan 3-4 minutes:

- ½ Vidalia or white onion, thinly sliced
- 1 Tablespoon extra virgin olive oil

ADD and cook for 5 minutes:

- 1 can pinto beans, drained and rinsed
- 1 can garbanzo beans, drained and rinsed
- 1 bag (12 oz.) frozen mixed vegetables
- 1 large can no-salt tomato sauce
- 1/3 cup water
- 2 Tablespoons reduced sodium Worcestershire sauce
         OR 1 Tablespoon Bragg Liquid Aminos
- 1 teaspoon cumin
- 1 teaspoon black pepper

CRUST:

- Use a corn muffin mix such as "JIFFY" and mix according to directions (1 JIFFY corn muffin mix, 1 egg, and 1/3 cup milk)

POUR vegetable and bean mixture into a 9 inch round or square baking dish. Top with corn muffin mixture.

BAKE at 400 degrees according to directions on corn muffin mix (about 15-20 minutes or until golden brown).

SERVES 6. This dish costs about less than $5 to make, or about 83 cents per serving.

TIP: You can bring the cost down even more by **planning ahead** to soak and cook dried beans instead of using canned beans. Once you learn what to do, it's easy. There are two ways to cook dried beans (one is quick, one is overnight). The directions will be on the bag. I have found the overnight method to be easier. Here's what I do: pour bag of beans into a large bowl, cover with plenty of water. Soak overnight. In the morning, drain the water, pour into a crock pot, add lots of water (if I have 2 cups of beans, I'll add 6-8 cups of water). Cook on low while you are at work.

Note from Nancy: Most Americans get far less than half the fiber they need. Using beans instead of meat in the Shepherd's Pie is a great way to reduce your bad fats ("saturated") and increase your dietary fiber. One-half cup of beans has 5-7 grams of dietary fiber. Aim for at least 28 grams of fiber every day.

GROWING HEALTHY KIDS TIP #20: Vegetables like zucchini, yellow squash, and carrots are "great to grate". **Teach your kids how to use the grater.   It's a "grate" job for them!**

To get your daily dose of vegetables with a dash of fun, check out these ideas:

Add 1 cup grated carrots to your tomato sauce or pinto beans.
Add 1 cup of grated zucchini to your favorite lasagna recipe.
Add 1 cup of finely grated yellow squash to your favorite chili recipe.

CHAPTER 5

RECIPE SHOPPING LISTS

It's bizarre that the produce manager is more important to my children's health than the pediatrician.

~Meryl Strepp

SHOPPING LIST: Fabulous Fruit Shakes

_____ Blue Diamond almond milk (with 60 calories per serving)

_____ frozen fruit (blueberries, bananas, strawberries, mangoes)

_____ Bob's Red Mill ground flax seeds

_____ vanilla and cinnamon (optional)

SHOPPING LIST: Pecan Pancakes with a Burst of Blueberries

_____ pecans
_____ quick cooking oats
_____ vanilla
_____ sea salt
_____ honey or agave nectar

SHOPPING LIST: Super Oats

_____ Steel Cut Oat (we recommend Bob's Red Mill Steel Cut Oats)

SHOPPING LIST: Garden Pizza
_____ Baby bella mushrooms

_____ sun-dried tomatoes or Roma tomatoes

_____ fresh spinach, red and green peppers, onions, olives

_____ extra virgin olive oil

_____ fresh garlic

_____ dried basil

_____ dried oregano

_____ extra virgin olive oil

_____ tomato paste

_____ Tandoori Naan flat bread

_____ Mozzarella cheese

SHOPPING LIST: PB&Bs

_____ whole grain bread (such as Arnold's "Flax and Fiber" or

"Double Fiber" bread)

_____ Smucker's Natural Peanut Butter (Creamy or Chunky)

_____ bananas

_____ raisins

SHOPPING LIST: Wrap It!

_____ extra virgin olive oil
_____ red wine vinegar
_____ sea salt
_____ black pepper
_____ tomatoes (plum, cherry, or grape)
_____ cucumbers
_____ green bell peppers
_____ radishes
_____ red onion
_____ flat leaf parsley
_____ low-fat feta cheese
_____ oat bran pita bread (we like Toufayan Bakeries brand)

SHOPPING LIST: Hummus

_____ canned garbanzo beans
_____ tahini (sesame seed butter)
_____ fresh lemon juice
_____ fresh garlic
_____ extra virgin olive oil (optional: black olives)
_____ sea salt

SHOPPING LIST: Success Snacks

_____ dried cherries or cranberries

_____ pistachios, shelled

_____ walnuts

_____ Kashi Heart to Heart cereal w/oat flakes & blueberry clusters

_____ dark chocolate (we use the Xocai brand)

_____ zip lock snack bags

SHOPPING LIST: Favorite Tomato Sauce

_____ ripe tomatoes or 2 28-oz cans of whole, plum tomatoes

_____ extra virgin olive oil

_____ sea salt

_____ garlic

_____ red pepper flakes

_____ dried or fresh basil

_____ balsamic vinegar

_____ sun-dried tomatoes

_____ spaghetti (we like Barilla Whole Grain Spaghetti)

SHOPPING LIST: Pesto

_____ garlic

_____ walnuts

_____ parmesan cheese

_____ fresh basil leaves

_____ extra virgin olive oil

SHOPPING LIST: Pico De Gallo
_____ tomato

_____ red onion

_____ jalapeño pepper

_____ green pepper

_____ sea salt

_____ limes

_____ extra virgin olive oil

_____ fresh cilantro

SHOPPING LIST: Garden Quinoa

_____ quinoa

_____ low-sodium chicken stock

_____ sea salt

_____ black pepper

_____ frozen chopped, mixed vegetables such as peas, carrots, green beans, corn

SHOPPING LIST: Guacamole
_____ Haas avocado

_____ lime or lemon

_____ fresh garlic

_____ hot sauce (we like Crystal Hot Sauce)

_____ fresh cilantro

_____ sea salt

SHOPPING LIST: Mashed Cotatoes

_____ a head of cauliflower

_____ Fleishmann's Olive Oil spread

_____ skim milk

_____ sea salt

_____ black pepper

SHOPPING LIST: Frittata with Spinach and Cheese
_____ extra virgin olive oil
_____ an onion
_____ fresh spinach
_____ sun-dried tomatoes
_____ eggs
_____ extra sharp cheese
_____ freshly grated parmigiano-reggiano cheese
_____ sea salt
_____ black pepper

SHOPPING LIST: Veggie Sloppy Joes

_____ an onion
_____ garlic
_____ green pepper
_____ extra virgin olive oil
_____ Morningstar Farms Grillers Recipe Crumbles
_____ black pepper
_____ 1 can (8 oz) no-salt added tomato sauce
_____ ketchup (without high fructose corn syrup)
_____ Worcestershire sauce
_____ whole grain hamburger buns

SHOPPING LIST: Brain Power Burgers

_____ canned wild pink salmon

_____ canned albacore tuna

_____ Dijon mustard

_____ flat-leaf parsley

_____ small yellow onion

_____ egg

_____ sea salt and pepper

_____ bread crumbs

_____ nonstick cooking spray

SHOPPING LIST: Black Bean Quesadillas

_____ 1 can black beans

_____ mild salsa

_____ cheddar cheese

_____ whole grain tortillas (we like La Tortilla Factory's Smart and
Delicious Torillas)

TIP: Fruits and vegetables should be half the food on your lunch and dinner plates.

SHOPPING LIST: Pasta with Walnuts

_____ extra virgin olive oil

_____ yellow onions

_____ fresh garlic

_____ a fresh red pepper

_____ dried red pepper flakes

_____ walnuts

_____ fresh parsley

_____ whole grain penne pasta (like Dreamfield's or Barilla)

_____ sea salt

_____ fresh ground pepper

_____ Parmesan cheese

SHOPPING LIST: Veggie Shepherd's Pie

_____ Vidalia or white onion
_____ extra virgin olive oil
_____ 1 can pinto beans
_____ 1 can garbanzo beans
_____ 1 bag (12 oz.) frozen mixed vegetables
_____ 1 large can no-salt tomato sauce
_____ reduced sodium Worcestershire sauce OR Bragg Liquid Aminos
_____ cumin
_____ pepper
_____ corn muffin mix

CHAPTER 6

SUPER FOODS

Don't eat anything your great-grandmother wouldn't recognize as food.

~Michael Pollan

TWENTY SUPER FOODS to keep you healthy:

- ✓ Almonds
- ✓ Barley
- ✓ Beans
- ✓ Blueberries
- ✓ Broccoli
- ✓ Dark chocolate (Xocai brand is the "healthy chocolate")
- ✓ Extra virgin olive oil
- ✓ Garlic
- ✓ Greek yogurt (we love Cabot's)
- ✓ Kale
- ✓ Lentils
- ✓ Oats (I prefer "steel cut" oats are best because they are less processed than "rolled" oats)
- ✓ Onions
- ✓ Oranges
- ✓ Parsley
- ✓ Quinoa
- ✓ Spinach
- ✓ Tomatoes
- ✓ Walnuts
- ✓ Wild salmon

Here are seven reasons why super foods should be at the top of your family's shopping lists:

1. Super foods improve your blood pressure.
2. Super foods improve your blood fats and cholesterol.
3. Super foods protect you against cancer.
4. Super foods give you energy.
5. Super food whole grains, beans, and lentils are very high in dietary fiber and help fill you up so you don't overeat.
6. Super foods protect your memory.
7. Super foods help you sleep well.

CHAPTER 7

FAMILY SHOPPING LISTS

A is for Apple. F is for Fiber. Z is for Zucchini.

Eat your alphabet.

~Nancy Heinrich

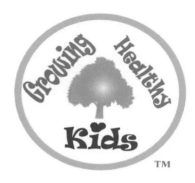

FRUITS:
- Apples
- Apricots
- Bananas
- Blackberries
- Blueberries
- Cantaloupe
- Cherries
- Grapes
- Grapefruit
- Kiwi
- Mangoes
- Oranges
- Papaya
- Peaches
- Pears
- Pineapple
- Plums
- Pomegranates
- Raspberries
- Starfruit
- Watermelon

VEGETABLES:

- Artichokes
- Asparagus
- Beets
- Broccoli
- Cabbage
- Cauliflower
- Celery
- Collards
- Corn
- Cucumbers
- Eggplant
- Green beans
- Kale
- Leeks
- Lettuce
- Lima beans
- Mushrooms
- Okra
- Onions
- Parsley
- Peppers (green, red, yellow, chili, banana, etc.)
- Potatoes
- Pumpkin
- Rhubarb
- Spinach
- Squash (yellow, green, butternut, acorn, spaghetti, Hubbard, etc.)
- Tomatoes
- Watercress

TIP: Aim for eating more vegetables than fruits each week.

BEANS AND LEGUMES:

- Black beans
- Fava beans
- Garbanzo beans (chickpeas)
- Great white northern beans
- Kidney beans
- Lentils (brown, yellow, red)
- Navy beans
- Pinto beans
- Split peas
- White beans

GRAINS:

- Barley
- Buckwheat
- Bulgur
- Millet
- Oats
- Quinoa
- Rice
- Rye
- Spelt
- Wheat

> **TIP:** Make at least half of your grains WHOLE grains.

NUTS AND SEEDS:

- Almonds
- Cashews
- Chia seeds
- Peanuts
- Pecans
- Pistachios
- Pumpkin seeds
- Sesame seeds
- Sunflower seeds
- Walnuts

ABOUT GROWING HEALTHY KIDS

Growing Healthy Kids, Inc. is a movement to educate and empower kids and adults about healthy eating and physical fun. This non-profit 501(c)3 organization creates innovative partnerships, programs, and products for global leadership in the prevention of childhood obesity, diabetes, cancer, and cardiovascular disease.

We design and deliver solutions for families, schools, churches, companies, and governments. We develop model programs scalable to national and global levels and welcome your interest, ideas, and collaboration.

Our focus is to halt, reverse, and prevent childhood obesity and obesity-related diseases such as diabetes, joint and bone disorders, and cancer. We are working to improve the health – and lives – of America's children.

This is the first book in the Growing Healthy Kids series. Stay tuned for our next book. To learn more about the Growing Healthy Kids movement, go to:

www.GrowingHealthyKids.blogspot.com

ABOUT THE AUTHOR

Nancy Heinrich is an epidemiologist, diabetes educator, teacher, and parent. She is the founder of Growing Healthy Kids, Inc., an organization and movement started as the result of her work teaching thousands of adults with uncontrolled diabetes and prediabetes what to eat and how to control, prevent, and reverse diabetes.

NOURISH AND FLOURISH is Nancy's second book. Her first book is Healthy Living with Diabetes: One Small Step at a Time (available at www.ourlittlebooks.com). She creates web-based educational courses and videos and other tools for preventing and controlling diabetes and obesity. She uses her extensive experience in disease control and prevention acquired while working with Florida Department of Health and American Red Cross to make a difference in the childhood obesity epidemic. She is a graduate of University of Alabama-Birmingham's School of Public Health and Florida Atlantic University.

In 2012 Nancy was recognized as the Woman of Distinction in the Healthy Living category by the Girl Scouts of Southeast Florida. The cover of this book is dedicated to the girls and women in the Girl Scouts.

To contact the author about conducting an educational workshop at your school or company and to receive your copy of 10 Tips to Prevent Obesity and Diabetes, please email: growinghealthykidsnow@gmail.com.